Tight

Vagina

Exclusive Factors That Causes The Vagina Of A Lady To Be Tight

Dr. Steve Ross David

TABLE OF CONTENT

INTRODUCTION

Vaginal dryness or snugness is a typical issue around menopause. It happens when the tissue of the vagina isn't very much greased up. It can cause difficult intercourse. A modest bunch of variables can influence vaginal dryness. Estrogen is the main hormonal impact on the soundness of the vulva and vagina. Low estrogen can add to dryness. Diet and the utilization of specific drugs additionally are significant elements. You can expect any meds that influence dry eyes and dry mouth to comparably affect the vagina.

Estrogen levels in the blood change during the month and follow a typical example to each feminine cycle. For ladies who are not on hormonal contraception, levels are most minimal in the days not long before the beginning of feminine dying. This low level in some cases can add to vulvar and vaginal dryness. Exceptionally low-portion hormonal conception prevention can add to dryness.

Ladies irritated by vaginal dryness ought to have an exhaustive conversation and test with their medical services supplier to decide the most probable reason for these side effects.

This book will help with showing all you need to know about Tight vagina.

NORMAL FOUNDATIONS FOR A TIGHT VAGINA AND HOW TO LOOSEN THINGS

What are a few normal basic reasons for a vagina being excessively close?

There are various justifications for why your vagina might feel more tight than expected and make you experience torment. Underneath we've recorded normal donors, albeit this rundown isn't comprehensive.

1.) Contaminations

Normal contaminations that can cause snugness of the vagina incorporate sexually transmitted diseases (physically sent sicknesses) and vaginal yeast diseases.

VAGINITIS: Conceivable fixing connected with Vaginal Contaminations

Vaginitis alludes to diseases of the vagina, coming about because of the unusual development of microorganisms and yeast in the vagina.

Vaginitis makes a huge number of visits to the specialists' offices consistently in the US.

The most widely recognized type of vaginitis in ladies is a yeast disease, which are contagious contamination that normally results from the life form Candida. This issue might cause serious tingling in the genital region, bothering, copying, irritation, vaginal expansion, thick vaginal release, and that's only the tip of the iceberg.

The irritation that can result from contamination in the vagina can add to it turning out to be progressively close. It is essential to get tried and appropriately analyzed by a medical services professional so your vaginitis can be treated as quickly as time permits.

2.) Wounds or Actual Injury

Injury to the area or encompassing tissues from mishaps, actual injury, labor or unpleasant sex can be contributing variables. Also, those wounds causing scar tissue might represent extra difficulties.

3.) Dyspareunia

Dyspareunia is the clinical term for torment during penetrative sex coming from mental or actual issues. Dyspareunia can go before sex or happen during sex itself. Over the long haul, difficult intercourse can prompt a protecting reaction, causing the vagina to feel excessively close or disallowing infiltration.

Dyspareunia is a term depicting excruciating intercourse, where consistent genital torment happens previously, during, or after sex. This condition creates in numerous ladies and may result from different issues going from mental to physiological worries.

A lady with dyspareunia may have torment including entrance, trouble in utilizing a tampon, consuming or hurting torment, pulsating torment that goes on for a really long time even after sex, and a lot more issues.

These side effects can happen from any of the following:

• Vaginismus (muscle fixing)

• Wounds and additional injuries

• Irritation and contamination

• Vulvodynia, vulvar vestibulitis, and so forth.

• Medical procedures or explicit clinical therapies like pelvic radiation therapy for malignant growths

• Profound variables (injury, mental issues, stress)

On the off chance that you are managing tenacious agony from sex, it is fundamental to see your doctor to analyze the issue and treat it appropriately. Pelvic floor treatment can some of the time help you more than your primary care physician in the event that it is a strong issue.

4.) Changes to the Vaginal Tissues Post-Labor

Having kids vaginally can bring about changes to the flexibility and responsiveness of the vaginal channel along with actual changes to the muscles engaged with conceiving an offspring.

For other new moms, changes in estrogen levels while breastfeeding can cause vaginal dryness, bringing about uneasiness and some of the time loss of versatility. In different cases, scar tissue after birth could cause limitation of the pelvic floor itself.

5.) Vaginismus

Vaginismus is set apart by compulsory muscle fits happening only preceding infiltration. These fits can be both difficult and humiliating, emerging before sex, the Inclusion of a tampon, or during clinical assessments.

At the point when the vaginal muscles fit or choke automatically from the entrance (tampon, penis, sex toys, and so forth), it is called vaginismus, which might prompt trepidation and aversion of sex in ladies.

Ladies with vaginismus have portrayed their penetrative sexual encounters as feeling like the penis is "reaching a stopping point." A lady with this condition can have uneasiness and inconvenience while utilizing a tampon, or trouble going through a pelvic assessment.

These side effects can't be controlled without legitimate treatment. Vaginismus' accurate reason is obscure, yet it is frequently connected with mental factors like apprehension about sex and nervousness.

6.) Sexual Maltreatment Or Attack

Sexual maltreatment of any kind or degree is a damaging occasion that frequently lastingly affects the emotional well-being of the person in question. This can make sex-even consistently, consensual sexual experiences distressing and overpowering. Furthermore, as an actual response, the body's own "flight or battle" instrument might cause compulsory fixing of the pelvic floor muscles, prompting difficult intercourse or powerlessness to accomplish infiltration.

7.) Menopause And Hormonal Changes

Hormonal changes because of ailments, drugs, or menopause sometime down the road can bring about a scope of side effects including yet not restricted to vaginal decay, diminished flexibility of the vagina, dryness (less normal grease), mind-set changes, weight gain, and that's only the tip of the iceberg.

Ladies in their 40s and 50s by and large experience menopause, denoting the finish of their period and regenerative years. During this state, ladies might encounter hot glimmers, vaginal decay, weight gain, eased back digestion, diminishing of the hair, unpredictable periods, vaginal dryness, and extra changes. With diminished degrees of estrogen, this makes vaginal tissues slight, diminished vaginal grease, and loss of vagina stretch, which is called vaginal decay. There may likewise be a shortening and limiting of the vaginal waterway.

Vaginal decay is a pervasive justification behind difficult sex in a lady's midlife. Menopause causes tight vaginal muscles that cause aggravation, disturbance, tearing, and draining of the vaginal tissue while having penetrative sex, or when any infiltration happens. Diminished sexual well-being might result. Convey the progressions in your body to your primary care physician, so these side effects can be observed. Your OB-GYN might exhort medicines including a vaginal dilator, oils, pelvic floor works out, and hormonal treatment.

8.) Ailments, Treatment or Drugs

A few ailments, medicines, and conditions can bring about a fixing of or a failure to effectively 'relax'. Malignant growth therapies, for example, radiation, conditions that arouse or disturb encompassing tissues, and drugs that influence chemicals can all cause issues.

Having a tight vagina is a troublesome and normally ignored issue with regard to ladies' well-being.

A few worries might surface from vaginal snugness that can prompt various issues going from trouble in embedding a tampon to keeping away from gynecological assessments, or potentially in any event, having a difficult and beating sexual coexistence down.

It very well may be trying to examine, nonetheless, it is critical to realize that you are in good company and there are reasonable arrangements which can assist with loosening up vaginal snugness.

There are many reasons that add to vaginal snugness, however it is basic to comprehend the reason why your vagina is tight, and also track down viable strategies to treat it. Clinical experts by and large suggest vaginal dilators as one of the principal types of treatment.

9) Disease Treatment

Ladies who go through pelvic radiation for the therapy of tumors might have unfavorable well-being results that cause difficulties in their vagina.

By and large, a symptom of pelvic radiation is vaginal stenosis, which is characterized as unusual fixing and shortening of the vagina because of the development of scar tissue.

As the vaginal tissues recuperate from the pelvic radiation, scar tissue creates all through the vaginal wall and pelvic floor. Not in the least does this prompt the walls of the vagina to foster unbending nature and firmness, however it likewise causes shortening or limiting of the vagina.

This all adds to a deficiency of versatility and expanding snugness of the vagina, keeping ladies from performing ordinary errands, for example, embedding a tampon, going through pelvic assessments, infiltration of items (eg: sex toys), and sex. It is shown that most specialists suggest utilizing a vaginal dilator after your pelvic radiation therapy to lessen the gamble of contaminations.

10) Labor

Labor sadly can negatively affect a lady's body.

Each pregnancy shifts and there are physical and mental variables that influence your body. Besides the fact that a lady encounters serious irritation levels in her vagina and pelvic district after labor, however it is normal to likewise foster scar tissue all through the vaginal walls and pelvic floor.

This scar tissue can bring about a reaction to C-Areas, or episiotomies, where the vagina is sliced during labor to make the conveyance of the child simpler. Tears coming about because of conveyance can likewise add to the advancement of scar tissue, which causes the vagina to feel tight.

There are numerous post-pregnancy gives that can happen like diminished pelvic floor strength, excruciating sex, vaginal snugness, vaginitis, irritation, touchiness, vaginal dryness, and that's just the beginning. It is essential to address any post-pregnancy issues that your body is encountering with your OB-GYN and a pelvic floor actual specialist.

11) Pelvic floor muscles

Your pelvic floor muscles can turn out to be agonizingly solid and make the region around the vagina tight.

These are the muscles that we use to control our bladder and solid discharges. At the point when these muscles are exhausted, they begin to hold an excessive amount of pressure.

The mind might see any outer boost as a "danger," which can cause fixing of the pelvic floor muscles that fold over the vagina and in this manner strongly close it. Throbs in the pelvis can transform into anguishing issues and fits. This can make the powerlessness to have penetrative sex, pelvic assessments, and even trouble embedding a tampon.

Tight pelvic floor muscles can cause crippling and sharp agonies that shoot all through the vagina or entrail, going on for hours or days. Specialists suggest treatment which for the most part incorporates vaginal dilators.

HOW MIGHT I DECREASE MY VAGINAL SNUGNESS?

Albeit each lady's body and vagina is special, a few dependable strategies can be integrated into your routine to assist with diminishing the side effects and fundamental reasons for feeling excessively close.

1) Use a Dilator To Assist with extending The Vagina

One of the best, solid, reasonable, and least difficult ways of doing this is utilizing an extraordinarily planned vaginal dilator.

Clinical experts quite often suggest vaginal dilators as a strategy for successful treatment for every one of the circumstances recorded over that add to vaginal snugness. It is vital to speak with your PCP to recognize and analyze the progressions happening in your vagina.

What is a Vaginal Dilator?

A vaginal dilator is a clinical gadget formed to look like a tampon or dildo tenderly tightened towards the inclusion highlight make starting infiltration more straightforward. They are produced using clinical level materials designed to be agreeable and delicate on the encompassing tissue and are accessible in a wide scope of sizes and lengths.

Numerous basic ailments adversely influencing the flexibility of the waterway can be tended to with a vaginal dilator. Those conditions might incorporate difficult sex, vaginismus, vaginal stenosis, vestibulodynia, vulvodynia, menopause, vaginal torment, and orientation attestation.

Vaginal dilators are tube formed gadgets that are utilized to increment vagina stretch and versatility. They come in various sizes changing long, outline, and width. The VuVa Attractive Neodymium Attractive Vaginal dilators were intended to mitigate pelvic and vulva torment in a patient who experienced sexual brokenness because of excruciating penetrative sex. The sizes range from 4-6.5 crawls long to 0.35-1.65 creeps in width. The cylinders are like the state of a tampon and make inclusion simpler with their tightened closes. It is more viable to utilize dilators that are firm plastic for the greatest stretch assuming that your muscles are exceptionally close, as opposed to silicone dilators.

How does a vaginal dilator function?

At the point when a vagina feels tight, a dilator tenderly releases and grows the vaginal opening and channel, permitting you to advance at your own speed and increment the size and length steadily as ease increments over the long run. There are numerous assets on our site on the best way to extend your vagina. Dilators train the vaginal muscles and tissues to unwind and extend, empowering blood stream and versatility to the area and quieting the related nerves during sex, for instance. Dilators likewise assist ladies with turning out to be mentally more alright with the thought and sensations of entrance, expanding their degree of solace at their own speed and individually in the protection of their homes. In general, this assists with expanding fearlessness and tranquility.

How to utilize vaginal dilators?

Utilizing vaginal dilators is exceptionally straightforward and should be possible at home. Whenever you have counseled a pelvic floor specialist and laid out the dilator size you ought to start with, it ought to be noticed that the use each day and week changes. We likewise have a video to assist you with picking your size.

1.   Guarantee that you designate time in your day to day daily practice to unwind and draw in with this cycle. It is ordinary to feel uneasiness while starting to utilize the vaginal dilators, be that as it may, it ought not to be difficult.

2.   Choose a confidential place where you won't be intruded.

3.   Pick the dilator with the smallest size or the size that has been prescribed to you by a clinical expert.

4.   Ensure the dilator is washed with cleanser and water. Air dry totally.

5.   For normal grease, utilize a water-based oil to cover the dilator prior to utilizing it.

6.   Recline (on a bed, seat, or couch), twist your knees and spread your legs completely open. In some cases utilizing a mirror might help in reviewing your vaginal entry.

7.   Begin by putting the tip of the dilator at the entry of the vagina and utilizing your breathing to effectively keep the pelvic floor muscles loose.

8.   Slowly and tenderly add the dilator. Leave the dilator in for the suggested time, and when you are agreeable, tenderly move the dilator in and out.

9.   Clean the dilator when every use with boiling water and cleanser. Dry completely.

As you develop more agreeable through training, you can expand the dilator size and the term of purpose. Guarantee that you talk with a clinical expert to direct and screen your state.

What's in store after widening treatment?

Widening treatment is a successful method for expanding the versatility of your vagina and eventually transforming you. It helps in reinforcing and settling the pelvic floor and vaginal muscles. Besides the fact that this assistance in lightens agonizing sex, however, it makes entrance simpler. You never again need to try not to utilize tampons or excuse pelvic assessments. Studies have shown that ladies worked on in sexual capability subsequent to utilizing vaginal dilators and that the dilators were viable in forestalling vaginal. Enlargement treatment can assist ladies with recovering their certainty and permit ladies to partake in typical exercises with decreased torment side effects.

How do vaginal dilators help?

Vaginal dilators assist with preparing the pelvic floor and vaginal muscles to unwind. The pelvic floor muscles protract around the dilators and reinforce the muscles, making them more adaptable and controllable. The general extreme touchiness that happens in the vulva and vagina is diminished by using vaginal dilators. By steadily expanding the size of the dilators, it permits you to work on unwinding and controlling your vagina and pelvic floor muscles. Since the human body creates its own attractive field, magnets can be utilized to reestablish and loosen up your pelvic floor. While utilizing Vuva dilators, the expansion of Neodymium magnets in the dilators builds the bloodstream to the vagina to balance illness and corrosiveness.

2) Use a Pelvic Wand To Assist with extending The Vagina

A pelvic wand is gainful for tending to muscle snugness, trigger focuses, and delicate focuses in the pelvic floor muscles. Also, the pelvic wand can be utilized for delicate preparation, myofascial delivery, and relaxing scar tissue around and inside the vagina.

How Does a Pelvic Wand Function?

For pelvic trigger point and delicate point torment, Close Rose pelvic wands are ideally suited for those hard to arrive at pelvic floor muscles, for example, obturator internus and puborectalis. The double end can be utilized rectally or vaginally. We much deal different sorts of wands-some that offer vibration and, surprisingly, on that can hold a hot or cold temperature!

Pelvic wands are frequently utilized cursorily for perineal back rub, introitus extending, and to arrive at more profound pelvic floor muscles. They are an incredible choice for anybody experiencing Endo/IC torment, tailbone torment, hypertonic muscles, or profound dyspareunia.

<u>All in all, what is better for pelvic torment; a vaginal dilator or pelvic wand?</u>

Contingent upon your particular conclusion and objectives, a pelvic wand or vaginal dilator might be suggested. Also, now and again, you could profit from both vaginal and pelvic wands to treat pelvic agony.

In the easiest of terms, vaginal dilators are utilized to treat limitations at the vaginal opening and trouble with any type of entrance, for example, from pelvic tests, tampons, or sex. They are Great for those with vaginismus, scar tissue, or hypertonic muscles.Pelvic wands are utilized cursorily for perineal back rub, introitus extending, and to arrive at more profound pelvic floor muscles. They are perfect for those experiencing Endo/IC torment, tailbone torment, hypertonic muscles, or profound dyspareunia.

As referenced above, pelvic wands and vaginal dilators frequently work fabulous together as a matter of fact, we call them pelvic torment major advantages!

What activities can help stretch and release the vagina?

Particular sorts of extending and activities can increment deliberate command over the muscle structure and tissues of the vagina. Personal Rose has numerous assets around pelvic floor stretches and activities to assist with loosening up the pelvic floor.

Frequently when we discuss pelvic floor works out, kegels practices ring a bell. Kegels are a constriction of the pelvic floor muscles and, at times, can make issues of vaginal and pelvic floor snugness more terrible and can increment torment. Thusly, Kegels ought to be kept away from until agony and limitation in the pelvic floor have been tended to.

STEP BY STEP INSTRUCTIONS TO FIX YOUR VAGINA NORMALLY

Ladies who carry on with life and do things like, indeed, have bodies, go through pregnancy, convey infants or experience menopause or regenerative medical problems will probably eventually encounter some level of vaginal laxity. What's more, can we just be look at things objectively, that is just pretty much we all. However numerous ladies don't examine the issue with their doctors since they feel humiliated or they are worried that the main choice for fixing the vagina is a medical procedure. Vaginal fixing isn't a vanity project. A solid vagina is critical to pelvic wellbeing and by and large wellbeing and bliss. Luckily there are a few simple, effortless, normal choices that ladies have tracked down effective in treating vaginal laxity, or detachment.

Reasons for Vaginal Laxity

Hormonal variances and actual strain or weight on the vagina and other pelvic organs can prompt vaginal laxity.

Normal causes include:

• Vaginal labor that stretches muscles, ligaments and vaginal walls

• Diminished estrogen levels brought about by menopause

• Decreased estrogen levels brought about by medical problems

• Maturing muscles and ligaments making a debilitated pelvic floor

• A lady's hereditarily resolved actual design

What are the Side effects of Vaginal Laxity?

Side effects of vaginal laxity can include:

• Vaginal dryness

• Vaginal torment or distress during intercourse

• Uncommon draining after sexual movement

• Absence of grease during intercourse

• Urinary incontinence

• Consuming during pee

• Unforeseen and pressing requirements to pee

• Incessant urinary plot contaminations

• Unusual vaginal release

• Consuming or tingling in the vaginal or vulvar regions

• Diminished charisma

• Absence of sexual excitement

• Decrease in sexual fulfillment during intercourse

Fixing Your Vagina Normally

Exercise, estrogen and spices can all assist diminish vaginal laxity with a little exertion consistently.

Kegel Exercise

Kegels are incredibly viable for conditioning the pelvic floor, diminishing incontinence and working on sexual fulfillment.

Kegels are fixing the muscles of your pelvic floor in a few arrangements of reiterations over the course of the day. Contemplate the muscles you would use to quit peeing - those are the ones you need to target. Nonetheless, while your pelvic floor muscles assist with supporting the vagina and encompassing designs, they are not what make up the vaginal walls. Still - having better tone and backing for your pelvic organs is all significant for vaginal wellbeing.

Estrogen Treatment

Chemical substitution treatment (HRT) used to be a kind of terrifying, sometimes good, sometimes bad treatment. Today ladies can have their HRT exceptionally formed and intended to suit their bodies, necessities and objectives. HRT replaces the chemicals the body no longer makes after menopause or when the body diminishes the development of estrogen and different chemicals for other clinical reasons.

HRT creams offer customization, adaptability and basic, simple use of chemicals that are then ingested through the skin and into the circulatory system. HRT cream permits the right portion of chemicals to be retained through the skin and into the circulation system to assist with easing hot blazes, night sweats, sadness and different side effects of menopause.

Natural Medicines

Natural creams and splash can be viable in treating vaginal laxity. Converse with your urogynecologist for suggestions to guarantee what you are utilizing is non-poisonous and ok for vaginal application.

What Doesn't Work

Vaginal fixing pills might flaunt every single regular fixing and commitment wonderful, long haul results, however they don't have the science to back up their cases - and they don't work. At times, these pills might try and be destructive - a lot of "regular" fixings can cause unfriendly responses.

Making the Following Stride

Assuming your inconvenience and side effects of vaginal laxity are steady, counsel your urogynecologist. In the event that your condition is serious, your urogynecologist might suggest a careful arrangement known as a vaginoplasty, which is utilized to treat outrageous extending, muscle detachment or tearing during labor. The medical procedure can likewise work on urinary incontinence.

diVa® laser vaginal restoration advances the development of new collagen structures, which fortify, firm and "stout" the vaginal walls. It likewise restores the vaginal coating to work on normal oil. diVa® is likewise used to help gentle instances of urinary incontinence.

23 REALITIES YOU OUGHT TO BE FAMILIAR WITH VAGINAS

Regardless of whether you utilize the term vagina to depict the life systems up in your jeans, it's all only one little piece of the enchanted occurring between your legs. In fact, your vagina is only the trench that runs from your vulva (the noticeable region that incorporates the internal and external labia, clitoris, and perineum) to the cervix (the lower piece of the uterus).

1. The Sweet Spot is a GD lie!

As per a new Cosmoinvestigation, a group of scientists formally begat the expression "Sweet spot" in the mid '80s. They named the thing, which they portrayed as a "delicate" "little bean," for German specialist Ernst Gräfenberg (no doubt, a fella). What's more, very much like that, your most baffling phony body part was conceived.

Many preliminaries utilized reviews, pathologic examples, imaging, and biochemical markers to attempt to pinpoint the slippery Sweet spot unequivocally.

"I don't think we have any proof that the Sweet spot is a spot or a construction. "I've never seen the motivation behind why it was interpreted as some new sexual organ.

You can't normalize a vagina — there is no consistency across ladies with respect to where precisely we experience joy."

For certain ladies, there is sexual responsiveness where the Sweet spot should be. In any case, for other people, there's none. Or on the other hand it's to one side. Or on the other hand it's in a couple of spots. Furthermore, that is somewhat the general purpose. It's all alright. It can all vibe great.

2. Not every person who has a vagina is a lady.

An individual's sexual organs are not a sign of their orientation, and it's unsafe to expect so. An individual brought into the world with a vagina may likewise distinguish as a trans man, male, non-twofold, genderqueer, orientation liquid, or orientation nonconforming.

3. Few out of every odd lady is brought into the world with a hymen.

That meager layer to some degree covering the entry to the vagina isn't ensured. Furthermore, regardless of whether you were brought into the world with one, playing sports as a youngster, utilizing tampons, or irregular operations can "break" it. So not having a hymen doesn't exactly mean you've never had intercourse.

4. Labia come in all shapes and sizes.

The labia, or the lip-like tissue around the kickoff of your vagina, can be just one-quarter inch or up to two inches wide, per ACOG. In this way, better believe it, each young lady is an exceptional and extraordinary unicorn.

5. Your vagina generally has a tad of yeast in it.

Regardless of whether you have an all-out yeast disease, your hoo-ha ordinarily contains a portion of the parasite. It's just when your microbiome, or the solid exhibit of microorganisms in your vag, gets upset by lubes or even anti-toxins that the yeast can congest and cause side effects like tingling and consuming, per ACOG.

6. The encompassing region frequently can be various tones.

The shade of your labia or vaginal tissue isn't really connected with the tone of the remainder of your skin. Some fair-looking ladies have brown or purplish labia, while a more obscure-cleaned lady can have a lighter vulva. You can have varieties in various regions — for instance, your labia could be on the more obscure side yet your perineum could be pale pink. Whatever your colorway, there's no "ordinary." She's ideal simply how she is.

7. Its walls are creased.

Normally, the walls of the vagina lie compacted against one another. However, the sides can isolate and broaden, similar to the way an umbrella opens. The vagina commonly grows to two inches wide during sex and it can get considerably greater to permit a child to go through it.

8. Bunches of sex won't extend it.

As made sense of over, the vagina is unimaginably versatile, so it generally gets back to its standard snugness after sex. So could we at any point all consent to kill the misogynist "sausage in a lobby" representation for eternity? Much obliged.

9. Nor will it recoil on the off chance that you go through a drought.

From the start, your vaginal muscles might be tense after weeks or month without sex or foreplay, yet infiltration ought not be difficult. Converse with your doc assuming it proceeds.

10. You can reinforce it like some other muscle.

Your pelvic floor muscles hold your vagina, uterus, rectum, and urethra set up, as per ACOG. So when your pelvic floor is feeble, you know, similar to just after you push a human out of you, holding your pee can be more diligent. However, doing Kegels can fortify the muscles encompassing your urethral and vaginal openings. Simply brace down as though you're halting the progression of pee, hold for three seconds then, at that point, unwind for three seconds. Complete 10 reps every day, moving gradually as long as 10-second holds.

11. It's overflowing with microscopic organisms.

The main bug taking up home: lactobacilli, a strain that produces lactic corrosive, which holds terrible microorganisms in line so you don't get a contamination. All things considered, kindly never under any circumstance put yogurt, which contains lactic corrosive (or any food), up in there. It won't fix yeast contamination and may prompt more issues.

12. It's self-cleaning.

Release flushes out cells from the vaginal wall, overabundance water, and microorganisms. At the point when you're in the shower, a straightforward swipe of gentle, fragrance free cleanser and water between the labial folds and along the perineum is all you want.

13. There are two significant reasons for vaginal torment.

Vaginismus, which makes the vaginal muscles contract automatically, can make it troublesome or difficult to have intercourse, utilize a tampon, or even go through a gyno test. It tends to be dealt with by means of non-intrusive treatment or directing. The other, portrayed by vulva agony, stinging, or responsiveness so extraordinary that immediate touch is difficult to bear, is vulvodynia. These are frequently analyzed after gynos preclude different circumstances, like a terrible yeast contamination. Antidepressants can frequently assist with decreasing the agony.

14. Its fragrance can change consistently.

It will in general be acidic before your period and impactful a while later. Your smell may be more observable post-exercise, on account of sweat organs, and during sex, because of the normal grease you produce. "Having a slight scent to your vagina is customary. "Regardless, when the fragrance significant solid areas for becomes, or is went with a weird delivery, this moment is the perfect open door to see the trained professional."

15. Climaxes are great for you.

Having ordinary sex (even with yourself) and climaxes can really assist with decreasing pressure and nervousness, says Dr. Boyle. "Climaxes increment estrogen creation, which increments oxytocin discharge and decreases cortisol [the principal stress hormone] creation."

16. In any case, a lot of sex can toss it messed up.

A lot of activity in a brief timeframe may leave you scraped or with a urinary parcel disease. Luckily, drinking additional liquids and peeing post-sex can keep a UTI under control.

17. Release changes all through your cycle.

However, your vag produces up to two teaspoons of flimsy, clearish release a day during ovulation, just before your stream it's creamier and thicker. "The adjustment of your release during ovulation establishes a neighborly climate for the sperm to head out up to the egg. In the event that it at any point tingles, consumes, smells foul, or seems to be curds, see your gyno.

18. Your vagina is certainly not a dark opening.

It's unimaginable for anything (like a tampon) to get lost up there since the cervix closes off access. However, in the event that a tampon gets far off, fish it out while crouching and pushing ahead. On the off chance that that doesn't work, your gyno can eliminate it rapidly.

19. Clits behave like faux pases when you're turned on.

Excitement makes your clitoris become engorged with blood and develop bigger.

20. Your vagina can be twofold in size.

Ladies' vaginas can change in size and shape when they're stimulated. Yet, because of a peculiarity called rising, it's absolutely feasible for your vag to twofold in size. This implies the upper 66% of your vagina grows, empowering sperm to effectively climb into the cervix more.

21. Your clitoris is far more touchy than a penis.

Perhaps it appears glaringly evident, yet there are 8,000 tactile sensitive spots in the clitoris, while the penis just has 4,000. That could make sense of why a clitoral climax is for the most part undeniably more extreme than a peen's.

22. Your vagina is comparably acidic as wine.

No, truly: The typical vaginal pH for vaginas is 3.8 to 4.5 and the pH of most wines fall around 3.0 or 4.0.

23. Vagina medical procedure is insanely costly and you most likely don't require it.

Vaginal methodology range from the G-shot (a collagen or filler infusion intended to expand the size of the much-discussed Sweet spot region) at around $1,500 to vaginal revival at around $7,000. These medical procedures are scarcely at any point covered by protection and are generally superfluous except if you have a real ailment causing you genuine clinical issues.

REALITY WITH REGARDS TO SEX AND VAGINAL FLEXIBILITY

A penis, regardless of how large, isn't sufficiently wide to loosen up a lady's vagina. Once again for individuals in the nosebleed segment?

Men, your penis doesn't pack sufficient power or bigness to loosen up the flexibility of a lady's vagina forever; thus, move past yourselves and stop skank disgracing physically open ladies.

Have you heard the saying?

Numerous men feel as though they can discover the nature of a ladies' yoni in view of how their penis feels when they are moving all through the vaginal trench of a lady, whom they are having intercourse with.

A portion of the legends related with a tight or free vagina:

1. Virgins have very close vaginas on the grounds that their hymen is unblemished.

2. Virgins ought to drain whenever they first engage in sexual relations.

3. Losing your virginity extends the vagina for all time.

4. Having a ton of sex with a solitary or having numerous accomplices will release the vagina.

5. Having a vaginal conveyance (labor) extends the vagina for eternity.

6. In the event that a lady is tight during sex, she has a quality vagina that hasn't been investigated by a great deal of men.

7. In the event that a lady's vagina is more loose during sex, she has been loosened up by man sexual accomplices and is in this way less attractive subsequently.

I recognize the conflict on ladies and our substantial independence, and for a really long time the thought has been that ladies ought to stay modest for one man to be commendable.

Certainly, western culture has developed from that old fashioned perspective, however the reality stays that ladies are still skank disgraced for having a sexual craving in an association with men. With a ton of spotlight being put on a lady's body count (the quantity of sexual accomplices she's had).

To do this actually, social fantasies encompassing vaginal snugness have arisen to check ladies' sexual transparency.

Storage space talk where folks say that sex wants to toss 'a wiener down a corridor' to drag a lady's worth through the mud assuming she's known to be...

COMPELLING HOME SOLUTIONS FOR VAGINAL DRYNESS

Numerous ladies could feel vaginal dryness eventually in the course of their life. Vaginal dryness is a typical issue that ladies might have a modest outlook on speaking with their PCPs. In any case, assuming it influences their regular routines, clinical assistance is important. An organ present in the belly (cervical organ) is liable for delivering regular oil in the vagina. It helps keep the vagina soggy and clean. Factors like a few prescriptions, a lessening in chemical levels, or breastfeeding can prompt the side effects of vaginal dryness. It can cause torment, consuming sensation, and disturbance when ladies take part in intercourse. Vaginal dryness can influence all ladies, yet it is more considered normal in menopausal ladies in their 50s.

On the off chance that you are somebody encountering vaginal dryness, you are in good company. So don't avoid getting clinical assistance. It'll assist you with having an agreeable existence.

The following are cures you can use at home to assist with vaginal dryness. These cures could assist you with dealing with the side effects and keep the condition from deteriorating. Prior to utilizing these natural cures, talk with your medical care proficient and get the vital conclusion.

1. Coconut Oil

You can utilize a characteristic oil, for example, coconut oil to help ease vaginal dryness.1 Virgin coconut oil is the regular oil got from mature coconuts. It has numerous medical advantages, and alleviating dry skin might be utilized. Coconut oil is a characteristic emollient (skin calming) and could help saturate the skin.4 You can apply coconut oil uniformly to the vagina by kneading gradually. Try to clean your hands first before you contact your reproductive organs.

2. Almond Oil

Sweet almond oil has been utilized to manage dry skin conditions by and large. Almond oil could give numerous advantageous impacts to the skin. It likewise has regular emollient property.5 You might utilize this normal home grown oil to help dispose of vaginal dryness.1 First, clean your hands. Almond oil can be applied around the vagina to dispose of vaginal dryness. Ensure your vagina is spotless and dry before you apply oil.

3. Olive Oil

Olive contains vitamin E, which is really great for keeping up with and further developing skin hydration and expanding its water holding limit. Loss of water from the skin surface is related with the skin layer called the layer corneum.6 Loss of water can make the skin dry. Olive oil may be helpful in getting alleviation from dry skin.1 Take some olive oil and back rub it in and around the vagina. You really want to clean up first before you apply the oil.

4. Soy

Soy contains synthetic mixtures which have numerous medical advantages. Dietary supplementation with soy may be useful in further developing menopausal side effects like hot glimmers and vaginal dryness, yet more examinations are expected to help its use.7 You can add soy and soy items to your food varieties and dishes to get the advantages.

5. Vaginal Creams

You can attempt a vaginal cream to assist with vaginal dryness.1 Utilizing a vaginal lotion can assist you with securing in dampness in and around the vagina and help in managing vaginal dryness. These lotions are as a rule of two kinds, inside and outside. Interior creams are embedded inside a vagina. Outside vaginal lotions are utilized for the vulva (the external piece of the female genitals).8

6. Water-Based Greases

You might utilize any water-based grease before intercourse to dispose of vaginal dryness. These greases could give present moment moisturisation.1,3 Oils may be applied in and around the vagina or on your accomplice's penis to keep away from any uneasiness during sex and help dispose of vaginal dryness.

7. Attempt Foreplay Before Sex

Vaginal dampness during sex relies upon excitement. Prior to enjoying sex, attempt more broadened foreplay. Appreciating more foreplay could assist you with getting more stimulated during sex and assist with forestalling vaginal dryness. Bartholin's organ present at the entry of the vagina produce dampness during sexual arousal.

8. Stay away from Scented Items

Try not to utilize vigorously perfumed cleanser, chemical or moisturizer in and around your vagina. These synthetics can make disturbance and lead dryness of your vagina. Continuously use fragrances free cleansers and moisturizers for your vagina. Utilizing perfumed cleansers, douches, or cleaning agents for your vagina is one of the elements answerable for causing vaginal dryness.3

However, there are concentrates on that show the advantages of the given home cures in managing vaginal dryness, these are deficient. There is a requirement for huge scope human investigations to lay out the genuine degree of the advantages of these home cures on human wellbeing. Hence, these ought to just be taken with alert and never as a substitute for clinical treatment.

What Causes Vaginal Dryness?

More often than not, vaginal dryness results from diminished levels of the female chemical called estrogen. Vaginal dryness can likewise foster in individuals going through treatment for another condition. A few normal reasons for vaginal dryness are:

- Breastfeeding

- Labor

- Assuming that you're on anti-conception medication pills

- Menopause

- Having your ovaries taken out

- Assuming you are getting treatment for disease, including chemotherapy or getting hormonal treatment

- Assuming that you are on enemy of estrogen medicine (used to treat endometriosis or uterine fibroids)

- Meds like allergy medicines (against unfavorably susceptible utilized for bothersome eyes or runny nose treatment) or antidepressants

- An immune system problem is called Sjogren's disorder. This problem can cause dryness in the entire body.

What To Be Familiar With Vaginal Dryness?

• Around 17% of ladies matured 18-50 experience vaginal dryness.

• Smoking can expand the gamble of vaginal dryness.

• Vaginal dryness can be a symptom of disease therapies, like radiation treatment.

• Normal sexual movement can assist with working on vaginal grease.

• Vaginal dryness can be a side effect of specific immune system problems, like lupus.

CONCLUSION

A few ladies could feel humiliated to converse with their PCPs about vaginal dryness. All things considered, vaginal dryness is a typical condition, and numerous treatment choices are accessible. You can contact your medical services supplier if:

•	You notice draining or any uncommon release from your vagina

•	You experience vaginal dryness for a really long time, and the home cures are not working out

•	The vaginal dryness is influencing your day to day exercises

•	You notice vaginal in the middle of between your periods or after you have engaged in sexual relations

You should not depend on home cures alone for the administration of vaginal dryness and ought to counsel a specialist for any exhortation in the event that the side effects don't improve with home cures.

Vaginal dryness can influence any lady, however menopausal ladies in their 50s are more inclined to it. This side effect is very normal, and numerous ladies face it eventually in their lives, so make it a point to clinical assistance on the off chance that it influences your day to day exercises. Also, there are a few things you can do at home to manage dryness in confidential parts. For instance, utilizing regular home grown oils like coconut, olive, or almond oil could assist you with disposing of vaginal dryness. In any case, these ought to be utilized in the wake of talking with a medical care proficient. Likewise, on the off chance that you feel any bothering in the wake of utilizing home cures, stop its use and connect with a medical services proficient.

Try not to allow humiliation to impede you of living a more joyful and more agreeable life.